I'm Not Really Seventy

Jake Adie

jadie
BOOKS

Published by
Jadie Books Limited 2007

ISBN 978 0 9549354-9-8

Cover illustration by Ian West

Typesetting by Jake Adie

Printed & bound by
York Publishing Services Ltd
64 Hallfield Road
Layerthorpe
York
YO31 7ZQ

For the not so young,
not so middle-aged,
not so sure

Other Not Really Titles

I'm Not Really 18 (female edition)
I'm Not Really 18 (male edition)
I'm Not Really 30 (female edition)
I'm Not Really 30 (male edition)
I'm Not Really 40 (female edition)
I'm Not Really 40 (male edition)
I'm Not Really 50 (female edition)
I'm Not Really 50 (male edition)
I'm Not Really 60 (female edition)
I'm Not Really 60 (male edition)
I'm Not Really 70 (female edition)
I'm Not Really Pregnant
I'm Not Really Getting Married
I'm Not Really Moving House
I'm Not Really Retiring
It's Not Really Christmas

Me Seventy?

I beg your pardon? Me? Seventy? Do you realise who you are addressing, my dear boy? A mere youngster in the prime of his life cannot, repeat, cannot simply metamorphose into a septuagenarian overnight. Let me be absolutely clear on this, my lad, I have never resembled a seventy-year-old in any shape or form whatsoever and have no intention of doing so at my time of life. And listen to me a moment, the fact that I have enjoyed in excess of three score years and nine really has nothing to do with the issue. For goodness' sake, time is too precious and life too short to waste on wandering around with a permanent *you-don't-know-how-well-off-you-are* expression on your face. Besides, septuagenarians have been around for as long as I can remember and they've always been different from me. I've never had any trouble recognising them at a hundred paces. In fact, it wouldn't surprise me if some of the poor old boys weren't well into their eighties, or even nineties by now. Furthermore, I've always considered myself a champion of the younger generations (not that I'm very much different in age, you understand). Mmm, have nothing but the utmost respect for them. After all, we slightly

more mature
folk should bear
in mind the
immensely more
complex
lifestyles with
which they have
to contend.
Totally baffling,
if you ask me.
None of your
simple
household
chores we grew
up with.
Polishing the
brass, scrubbing
out the scullery,
helping sweep
the chimney.
None of that in

my day. No, poor young encumbered folk these days have to endure a whole host of confusing routines to achieve the simplest of results: wireless telephone receivers, computerized washing-up machines, centrally-heated motor cars; what is the world coming to? But, you see, it isn't so very difficult for someone of my relatively tender years to adapt to modern technology and, in the process, qualify, quite easily, for acceptance within the ranks of society's younger contingent. You've only to take a look around my bungalow to appreciate my point: the very latest in music

cassette players
instead of an
SYO's twelve-
inch vinyl record
player; state-of-
the-art twin-tub
washing
machine – not a
mangle to be
seen and a
beautiful, up-to-
the-minute,
avocado green
bathroom suite
instead of old-
fashioned white
enamel. So, you
see, it is quite
unthinkable to
include me in
their number

regardless of the somewhat academic question of the number of years of my tenure on this planet. Anyway, if I really were a member of their club I'd be safely tucked away in one of those ghastly . . .

You see, if I am at liberty to enjoy life in my own home and mix as I please in the community without having to ask Matron for permission to hobble along to the High Street to procure this month's edition of some inept OAP periodical, I do not qualify in any shape or form for inclusion amongst their

Care Homes

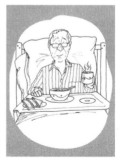

ranks. You are aware, I trust, of the mandatory requirement for citizens of due seniority to be installed into one of these hideous, institutional residential care homes. A euphemism if ever I heard one. Preposterous places. Let me tell you, it isn't common knowledge but the staff in these places are especially trained to behave as though the residents actually have control of their senses. To treat them as though they understand what they are doing when, in reality, as you and I know perfectly well, they certainly do not. Well, after all, their brains, or what's left of them, are nearly three-quarters of a century old. How could they know what they are doing? But that is not really the point, is it? Who gives a damn whether old arthritic Fred knows what he's doing? As long as he thinks he does, that's all that matters, surely. Look here, I'm not trying to be deliberately awkward or obtuse about this but the fact is these naïve, empty-headed, patronising little busybodies who masquerade as care staff have about as much substance between their ears as two lengths of freshly sawn softwood. So who is it precisely who is lacking in the grey matter stakes, mmm? Frauds the lot of them. Unable to procure worthwhile employment elsewhere, the miserable little madams think they can just trot along to the nearest OAP institution and bolster their failing confidence by bossing around a bunch of poor old SYOs who deserve to be treated with a good deal more respect. My goodness me, if I had my way I'd give them all a jolly good clip round the ear. That might install a sense of common decency into them. Anyway, you'll appreciate that I can't possibly be on the verge of joining forces with our humble SYO folk if only for the fact that I am able to facilitate a sufficient number of marbles to understand and elucidate this sorry state of affairs so objectively. Your average SYO would simply be unable to grasp the complexity of the situation. A person with any less an IQ would fail miserably to see through the hoodwinking that is clearly taking place here. In fact, I can tell you exactly the type of people they could do with in these so-called

care homes. Yes,
now I come to
think of it, I've
the perfect ones
in mind. You
see, since I've
not been feeling
quite myself
these past few
weeks, these two
young ladies
from along the
road have been
very kindly
calling on me to
carry out all
sorts of useful
errands. A great
boon, I'll have
you know.
They've been

taking care of my shopping and all manner of cleaning and household duties that I've really not been up to. And the wonderful thing is, they won't hear about taking a penny from me. Now how comforting and reassuring is that? Perfect little angels, the two of them. Mind you, I really don't know how to approach them but I could do with a little help in their looking out for some less reputable members of our community who, I'm sure, have been, somehow, entering my property uninvited lately. You see, there have been a number of quite valuable items gone missing and I'm at a loss to know what to do about it.

Can't bear all the palaver of getting the local constabulary involved. However, I digress, we really must return to the matter of our SYO folk. And, you know, without wishing to be unkind, how could I become a member of their club when they insist on wearing those silly looking . . .

You see, without my wanting to appear, well, unduly trendy I suppose, I feel it is incumbent upon me to point out that to be acknowledged by my contemporaries as a genuine SYO I'd need to don the pre-requisite Harris tweed three-piece, plus-fours suit complete with gold fob watch and chain and, in the most

Clothes?

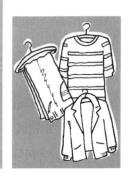

authentic of cases, matching eye monocle before even thinking about setting foot outside the front door. Not forgetting the calf-length worsted wool Argyles and suspenders. Oh, behave yourself! Not the type that, what do you call them?, cross dressers, that's it, the type that cross-dressers wear.

No, the ones that you sort of strap around your knees and hook on to the tops of your socks (which, take it from me, become extremely uncomfortable after a couple of hours). Anyway, I can excuse you if you are having trouble grasping the concept of life as an bona fide septy because, well, these poor old souls are just not normally-developed, modern, forward-thinking individuals like you and me. No, not in the slightest. The mere fact that we may have been around for a similar number of years is of little relevance. You mark my word, an awful lot more than out-of-date tweeds and the chalking up of three score years and ten is required to qualify as an authentic SYO. So, you will need to concentrate, I'm afraid. Which is not unreasonable because, and let us be absolutely frank here, there aren't many of their type around these days. Forgive me but most will have gone off to the great care home in the sky by now. (And, hopefully, taken their wretched dog-tooths with them.) Which, all in all, is fine by me because they'd be of precious little use to the likes of us youngsters if they were to have been left behind. No, if you've not been fortunate enough to witness the full splendour of sheer sartorial elegance when, for example, *I* step out for a brisk Sunday afternoon stroll in the park, you will not begin to appreciate the immeasurable contrast between me and the poor ageing folk whom we have chosen to consider in this tome. So, for those of you so disadvantaged, I will assist in portraying as graphic an image as will be possible within the confines of this chapter. Are you ready? Now, in place of the customary tweed hacking jacket you'll find me sporting the very latest in zip-up, lovat green, lightweight windcheaters. Complete with up-to-the-minute ribbed, elasticised, knitted waistband and matching collar and cuffs. Hold on, I've not finished yet. And, without a plus anything in sight, you'll be most impressed to learn that a freshly-pressed pair of tailored, medium-grey slacks will be perfectly complementing my quite obvious athletic gait. And as a finishing touch, the spring in my step will be provided courtesy of two, high-technology, training plimsolls. (I believe the accepted term for this form of footwear, if, as I suspect, you are unfamiliar, is 'trainers'.) Quite revolutionary they are too. So, need I say more? You have, no doubt, got the message loud and clear by now and could no more relate a youthful individual like me with archetypal septuagenarianism than you could imagine the Queen queuing at the checkout in the local supermarket. And, if this doesn't convince you, maybe I should give you a little insight into the difference in our respective tastes in . . .

Music

If, of course, that doesn't come across as something of a contradiction in terms. Now don't get me wrong, my philosophy has always been one of 'live and let live'. You know, the art of accepting that others are fully entitled to an opinion irrespective of their having been deprived of the advances made by the

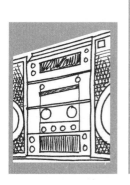

human race in subsequent, more recent times. Advances that will have rendered such thinking obsolete. That it may relate to an alternative, ancient culture whose people were unknowingly hindered by outmoded, arcane principles has little to do with the matter in hand. In a right and just society it is the duty of each modern-thinking citizen to exercise both tolerance and humility when considering any notable differences. Do you not agree? Of course you do. Young, agile-minded folk like you and me should, in the very least, set ourselves up as no less than characters of virtue and honour making due allowance for the inevitable flaws we will be apt to acknowledge in others born into less fortunate, less cultured generations. It is the very least we can do as a sign of respect for our forefathers. And a practice we should take utmost care to see is maintained at all times. You understand the importance I place on maintaining a respect for a people for whom we should all feel greatly indebted. So, when it comes to be that I should choose to take a little time out to sit back in my favourite recliner and relax for the odd half-an-hour beside the radiogram it will not be for the purpose of desensitising my considerable artistic faculties with the sort of inept, mind-numbing dross that is likely to set a septuagenarian's foot tapping. Please, do you mind? Credit me with some cultural aptitude. However, without wishing to appear unduly in accord with the latest our modern society

Music

has to offer in the world of aural sophistication, I have to admit that my ears are quite simply, automatically attuned to whatever constitutes cutting edge development where the subject of music is concerned. Nobody will ever hear me utter such time-dishonoured phrases as,

"That is not what *I* call music". Or, "For God's sake, you can't even hear the words he's singing". No, I simply move with the times. Allow my natural aptitude for recognising real, often, uncharted social issues expressed through modern diatonic, or otherwise, means. And if it's good enough for the generations entrusted by a rapidly ageing society to take responsibility as the nation's future custodians then it's more than good enough for me. And it is with this thoughtful, almost anthropological philosophy in mind that I am able to access the true depths of emotion, available exclusively to those with sufficient youthful, artistic mental agility, within the rich harmonic structure of a modern Beverley Sisters cassette recording. It would, of course, be presumptuous of me to expect you to have the same level of appreciation but, forgive me, I only wish to demonstrate my clear non-qualification status as an SYO. And I trust you are suitably convinced. But in the unlikely event that you are not, please allow me to place the question beyond any reasonable doubt by examining the matter of . . .

Sex

Not that there's ever been anything terribly simple about the subject. All things but, if you ask me. Root of all evil, if the truth be known. If you want my opinion, I believe the world would be a far better, more peaceful place to live in if it were banned tomorrow. Like religion. And money. And politics. As far as

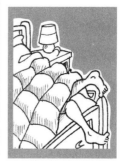

I'm concerned no good has ever been known to come out of any of them. Okay, I admit, there would be certain impractical connotations were sex to be removed from the agenda. But, in the case of SYOs, it is probably why they are a little better off than the rest of us. Mmm? I mean, without being burdened with having to perform the task with the required regularity over the years life must have been considerably less demanding. One of the world's more profound mysteries, don't you think? Well surely, we can all agree that the idea of them ever, well, you know, ever doing it is beyond comprehension. I mean, just look at them. Can you imagine? Of course you can't. They're just not designed to cope with such responsibilities. Any sane person can see that. It's obvious. I can remember as a young man when, well, you know, when things started to happen to me. When all of a sudden there appeared to be more to life that kicking footballs and collecting postage stamps. When I first experienced the calling from above. Usually in the middle of the night while I was fast asleep. And then, in the morning, I'd be embarrassed that Mum was going to find out I'd been called. Messy business. Anyway, even way back then, I clearly remember thinking about the poor SYOs who, it was patently obvious, were not on the team sheet, so to speak. Not being called like me. Which was just as well because they'd have had no effective means of responding, would they? And they still don't today. You can see that. It simply isn't in their make up. All right, all right, I know it begs a rather difficult biological question concerning the emergence of the subsequent generation but I am afraid I am not the fountain of all knowledge. I can answer most questions but you'll have to accept that some are just beyond me. I haven't a clue how rockets work, for instance. Or

cable television.
Or osmosis. But
that doesn't
mean they don't
work, does it?
You just have to
accept that some
things are best
left to experts to
explain.
Anyway, back
the matter in
hand. A casual
glance in my
direction will
confirm to even
the least
intellectually
perceptive
amongst us that
I am made of

different stuff entirely. Stuff that has clearly enabled me to play an active part in meeting the demands of my maker. Demands that I have taken to be the responsibility of each individual to ensure that the continuation of the species is not compromised in any way. And, more than most, through thick and thin, I have made it my duty to carry the torch at the slightest opportunity. And have never been known to complain in the process. That's how people of my generation were brought up to approach important matters. To place the highest priority on representing both God and country before personal consideration. I suppose it is why I had the calling all those years ago. Why I was singled out as one of the chosen ones. And, as part of the greater plan, no doubt, I have been duly rewarded in more recent times with being relieved of my duties. Not that I asked for it, you'll understand. If required to do so, I would have been prepared to continue until no longer able to participate. But who am I to question the good Lord? If it is His wish that I no longer serve then so be it. Which, in a strange way, puts me in a very similar position to the poor SYO folk we've been discussing. But that is where the similarity ends, I promise you. A

bit like the
difference in the
way they take
their . . .

Holidays

Well, as we all know, they don't so much take holidays as get *taken* on holidays. While the rest of us spend eons planning the next trip to the destination of our dreams, our sad contingent of SYOs simply trot down to the collection point next to the post office and wait for the arrival of the designated convoy of 56-

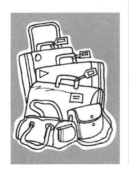

seaters each complete with flushing loo, semi-reclining seats and DDA-compliant loading platform. Yes, their idea of getting away from it all is to sandwich themselves in between 55 other variously assorted, but like-minded septys and have themselves transported at a steady 28.2 miles-an-hour around the British countryside by a PSV-licenced driver who has learnt enough about the heritage of at least one church, where and when a distant, long-forgotten TV celebrity spent their childhood plus a few grisly facts concerning who might have dismembered whom sometime during the fifteenth or sixteenth century in each village they are unfortunate enough to pass through. And given that the average SYO's memory retention is, at best, only partially effective for a maximum of three-and-a-half minutes from the point of input, our entire bus-load of happy holidaymakers

will be
physically
incapable of
recalling
anything
approaching five
percent of these
riveting facts
well before the
next settlement
comes into view.
Which is just as
well, when you
think about it,
because were
their minds to be
overcome with
inspiration at
having had their
knowledge bases
expanded to

such a degree, they'd be all but unaware that all available mind power is required to apply muscle control exercises to ensure that nature can successfully be put on hold until their arrival at the next scheduled market square public conveniences stop that is, hopefully, due to come on track just around the next double bend. Because, while the onboard flusher will, no doubt, handle the odd emergency adequately, coping with 56 simultaneous bladder crises would be stretching the designer's brief by a factor of several thousand. Of course, in an ideal world, there will be a motorway service area within muscle-clenching range enabling the driver to disgorge the entire contents of his mobile care module onto the tarmac of the designated coach park thereby allowing the tourists to systematically shuffle themselves into something mildly resembling a

human chain
before
embarking upon
the task of
gravitating, ever
so slowly,
towards, and,
subsequently,
away from, the
direction of the
multi-cubicled
wc facility. You
must have come
across them
yourself at
sometime. And
the memory of
such a sight will
enable you to
instantly
acknowledge the

vast chasm that exists between yours truly and these unfortunate, ageing folk. And if you care to exercise your powers of recall a little more energetically, you may recollect the sight of me and my good lady wife trundling along one of the overtaking lanes in our Morris Oxford heading for Eastbourne.

I'm Not Really Seventy

Yes, you read me correctly, Eastbourne, modern man's playground on the East Sussex Riviera. Where else, I ask you? Been going there for years. My God, it must be forty, or fifty by now. Started going with Ma and Pa shortly after the war when I was just a lad. Mind you that was long before they built those dreadful motorways where you've got, what do you call them, juggernaughts?, whizzing past on your left-hand side. There are no two ways about it, they should banned from the roads. Not like my day when they'd jolly well have to stay behind and curb any frustrations for not being allowed to speed up to forty- or fifty-miles-an-hour. However, please excuse me, I'm beginning to ramble. Goodness me, if I'm not careful, you might even start thinking I'm turning into an SYO myself. Banish the thought immediately. Anyway, it would be incomprehensible to relish the idea of me partaking of, for example, their types of . . .

Can you imagine anything more absurd? In fact, I wouldn't be too surprised to learn that our respective diets would fail to address the basic nutritional requirements of our individual generations. Not unlike differences that may naturally occur between two entirely separate species within the animal kingdom.

Food

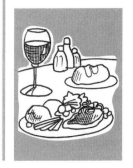

You're, no doubt, familiar with the term, one man's meat is another man's poison. Well, it had to derive from somewhere. All right, I may be exaggerating a little but you see what I'm getting at, surely. It isn't that I'm unsympathetic to their plight, you'll understand. And I fully accept that it's not their fault. It's just that they were introduced into this world during a totally different historical period. Take it from me, I know about such matters. You see, the kinds of foods available to current, younger generations bear little resemblance to the comparatively sparse, market garden-based produce to which their folk were restricted. I mean, it's quite obvious when you think about it, they weren't fortunate enough to have access to modern modes of transport that we simply take for granted today. Such as refrigerated container ships able to deliver exotic Far Eastern foodstuffs to our shops in so fresh a condition that we could be forgiven for mistaking them for freshly-picked, home-grown produce. This is what being a youngster like you and me means in this ecologically-friendly, global farming age. But spare a thought for our poor, deprived SYOs who did not have the good fortune to grow up with the benefits of such high technological advances just a brief 4x4 drive away. And 24-hours a day at that. The subject of sustenance will seem a wholly different proposition to them and one that will offer little hope of competing with, not just the variety of ingredients available to us, but the state-of-

the-art, four
North Sea gas
burning ring
technology we
have at our
disposal for food
preparation.
And,
furthermore,
you'll appreciate
how difficult it
must be for their
kind to come to
terms with the
strange labelling
that confronts
them each time
they peruse the
supermarket
shelves while we
feel perfectly at

home. I ask you, why are there no pop-in-the-microwave-for-three-minutes meals of tripe and onions for two? Or, pre-steamed, beef suet puddings in brown, mock take-away packaging ready to be transformed into instant meals within minutes of arriving home? Is this a fair way to treat a generation of folk who toiled their way through muck and bullets in no less than two world wars on account of our future well-being? Mmm? Not in my book it isn't. Not by a very long way. While we're spending a typical Saturday evening in our favourite restaurant enjoying the delights of prawn cocktail starters, mixed grill main courses and black forest gateau desserts should we not spare just a few moments to consider those of more senior years who will simply be unaccustomed, intimidated even, by the unfamiliar culinary terminology the rest of us use as part of our everyday language? And you'll notice I haven't even touched upon the subject of the drinks menu. Forgive me, please, but I doubt they've ever heard of, let alone sampled, a modern Riesling or Liebfraumilch. No, the limit of their gastronomic vocabulary starts somewhere around meat pie and ends firmly with brown ale. A million miles away from the world of culinary delights you and I take for granted. And, sadly, the picture appears all too familiar when you take a look at the way they approach their . . .

Hobbies

Oh dear, oh dear, what are we going to find here? SYOs and hobbies. Well, they're hardly synonymous with the subject, are they? I mean, hobbies are what you do when you find you have spare time on your hands, mmm? And what is it that SYOs have on their hands most of their waking hours? Yes, you've got

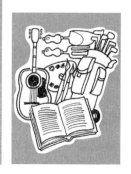

it, spare time. But have you ever witnessed an SYO even remotely involving himself in any kind of activity loosely resembling a hobby? No, me neither. It just isn't on their agenda. Unless we're both missing something. You never know. Could both be so wrapped up in our own lives, our own personal interests, that we simply fail to recognise what our fellow folk get up to. So, let's assume this is the case and examine the subject a little more closely. Right, where to start? How about taking a look at some of the common-or-garden pastimes available to us. Like, say, sky diving. No,

definitely un-
insurable. Or
windsurfing.
Erm? Could be
dodgy. Can't
imagine a septy
managing to
keep upright for
more than a
couple of
minutes let
alone climb on
board in the first
place. How
about hang-
gliding? No
chance of falling
off with all those
straps holding
you in. But
bowel control

could prove a bit problematic. Wouldn't fancy being in the vicinity myself. No, this is becoming futile. Let's try another, less energetic tack. How about jogging? Knee joints? Not exactly the most arthritic-friendly of pursuits. Swimming? Ehm, that sounds better. But, hold on, lung capacity?

Okay, what about rambling? Surely there can't be any form of physical exercise less demanding than strolling around the countryside upsetting farmers. Sorry, forgot about the stiles. All right, rowing? Another no-no. Climbing in and out of the boat just wouldn't work? Weightlifting? Silly. Goodness gracious, this is getting us absolutely nowhere. Perhaps it will help if we look at things from the opposite direction. I mean, by considering the likelihood of our trusty SYO becoming involved in the kind of hobbies I regularly participate in. Reasonable? If nothing else, it will further illustrate the yawning chasm between us and put this argument to bed once and for all. Okay, where to start? Ehm? Well, let's think. How about newspapers? No, perhaps that doesn't qualify. Shopping? Mowing the lawn? Sudoku? Oh God, what exactly *do* I get up to in my spare time?